AFTER THE BABY

Convert your favorite *baby* photographs (4" × 6") into beautiful and memorable *baby* announcement postcards.

Simply peel off the back of these self adhesive labels and paste them onto the back of the most precious photograph of your new *baby*.

Write your *baby's* vital statistics (i.e., weight, length, time of birth, etc.) on the postcards and send them to your friends and family to announce the arrival of your new bundle of joy.

Your friends and family will love receiving a photograph of your newborn *baby* along with your *baby* announcement.

For your convenience we have included a sample postcard to illustrate how practical and attractive these cards can *be*.

Produced by Elizabeth & Alex Lluch

Published by Wedding Solutions
© Copyright 1997

All rights reserved under International and Pan-American Copyright Conventions. No part of this book may be reproduced or transmitted in any form or by any means, electronic or mechanical, including photocopy, recording or by any information storage and retrieval system, without permission in writing from the publisher.

Printed in China

ISBN 1-887169-01-6

Sample Announcement

Complete this announcement with your newborn baby's information then simply peel and paste onto the back of your favorite baby photograph.

Place Postcard Postage Here

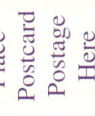

To:
Mr. and Mrs. Charles Hagler
353 Prospect St.
La Jolla, CA 92037

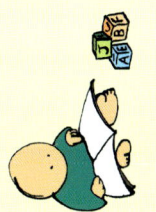

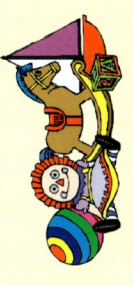

For U.S. Postal Service Use Only

© 1997 Wedding Solutions; San Diego, CA (619) 582-1878

Announcing The Arrival Of:

Name: Elizabeth Anne Burdell
Date: April 19, 1997
Time: 9:45 am
Weight: 7 lb. 4 oz.
Length: 19 inches
Proud Parents: William & Katherine Burdell

"Our New Bundle Of Joy!!"

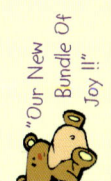

Sample Photograph

Send a copy of your favorite baby photograph (4"x 6") along with this unique and personal birth announcement!

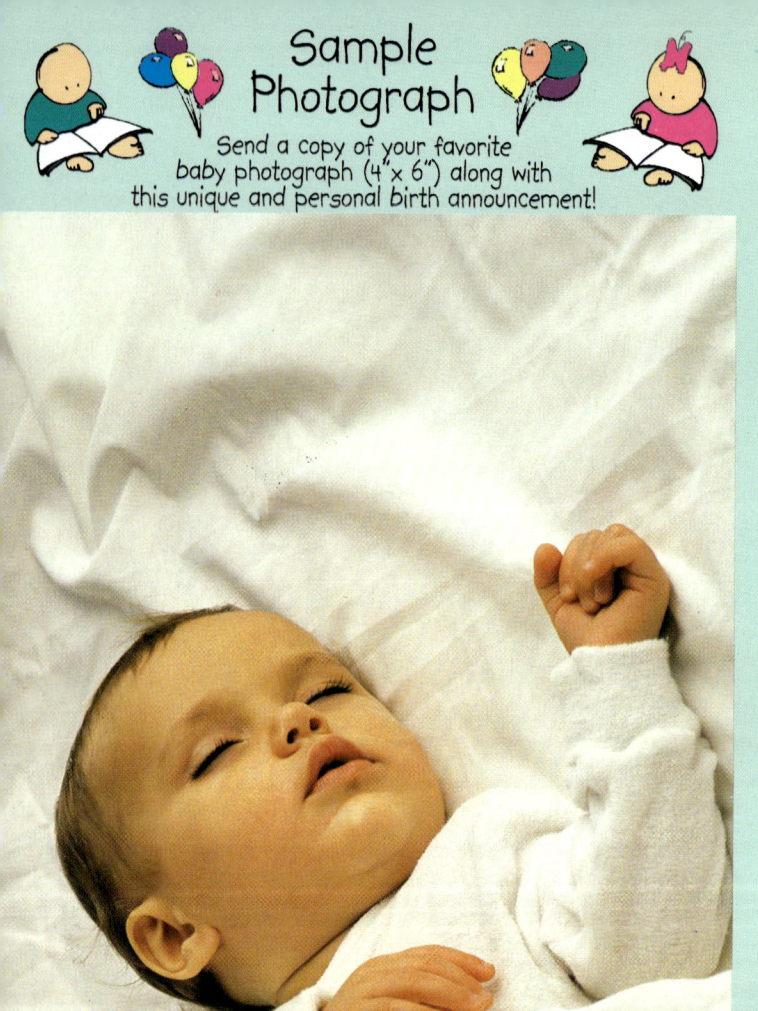

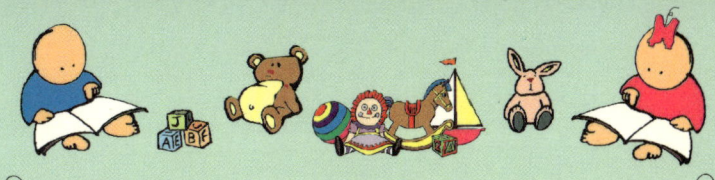

↶ Peel off label, then paste onto the back of your baby photograph. ↷

Place Postcard Postage Here	

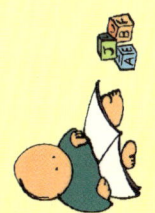

To:

© 1997 Wedding Solutions; San Diego, CA (619) 582-1878

For U.S. Postal Service Use Only

Announcing The Arrival Of:

Name: EDEN ELIZABETH PAGE EICHER
Date: Sept. 10, 2002
Time: 5:19 p.m.
Weight: 9 lbs. 13/4 oz.
Length: 20 1/2 in.
Proud Parents: Keith & Paula Eicher

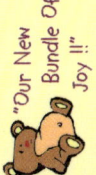

"Our New Bundle Of Joy!!"

↶ Peel off label, then paste onto the back of your baby photograph. ↴

Place Postcard Postage Here

To:

© 1997 Wedding Solutions; San Diego, CA (619) 582-1878

↶ Peel off label, then paste onto the back of your favorite new baby photograph. ↴

Announcing The Arrival Of:

Name:

Date:

Time:

Weight:

Length:

Proud Parents:

"Our New Bundle Of Joy !!"

For U.S. Postal Service Use Only

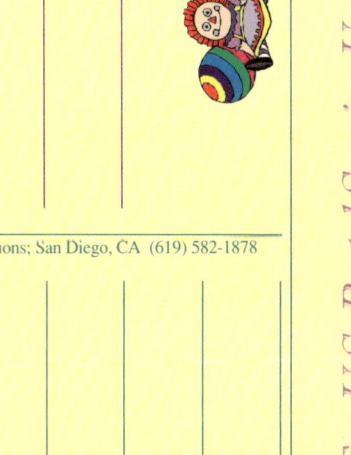

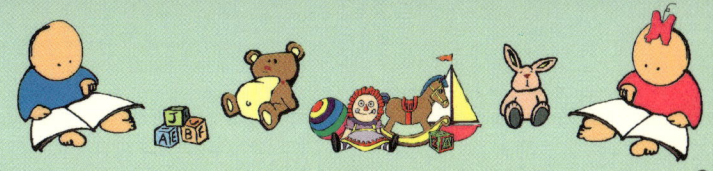

↳ Peel off label, then paste onto the back of your baby photograph. ↲

Place Postcard Postage Here

↶ Peel off label, then paste onto the back of your favorite new baby photograph. ↷

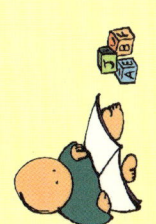

To:

© 1997 Wedding Solutions; San Diego, CA (619) 582-1878

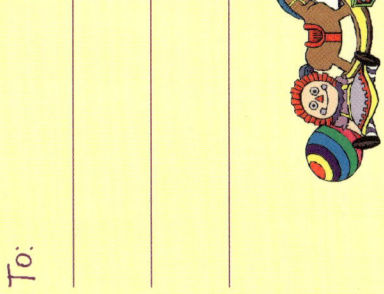

For U.S. Postal Service Use Only

Announcing The Arrival Of:

Name:

Date:

Time:

Weight:

Length:

Proud Parents:

"Our New Bundle Of Joy !!"

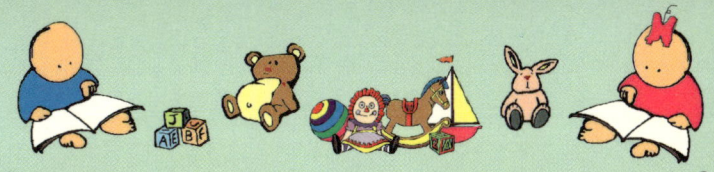

↳ Peel off label, then paste onto the back of your baby photograph. ↲

Place Postcard Postage Here

↶ Peel off label, then paste onto the back of your favorite new baby photograph. ↷

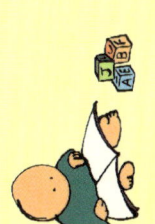

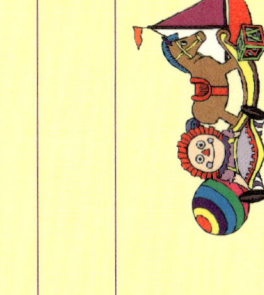

To:

© 1997 Wedding Solutions; San Diego, CA (619) 582-1878

For U.S. Postal Service Use Only

Announcing The Arrival Of:

Name:

Date:

Time:

Weight:

Length:

Proud Parents:

"Our New Bundle Of Joy !!"

↶ Peel off label, then paste onto the back of your baby photograph. ↷

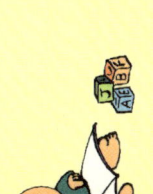
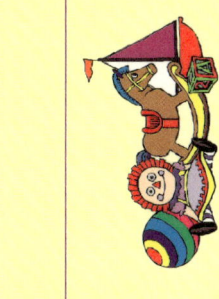

Place Postcard Postage Here

To: _____

© 1997 Wedding Solutions; San Diego, CA (619) 582-1878

For U.S. Postal Service Use Only

Announcing The Arrival Of:

Name: _____

Date: _____

Time: _____

Weight: _____

Length: _____

Proud Parents: _____

"Our New Bundle Of Joy !!"

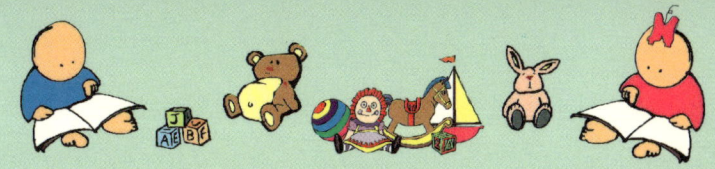

↪ Peel off label, then paste onto the back of your baby photograph. ↩

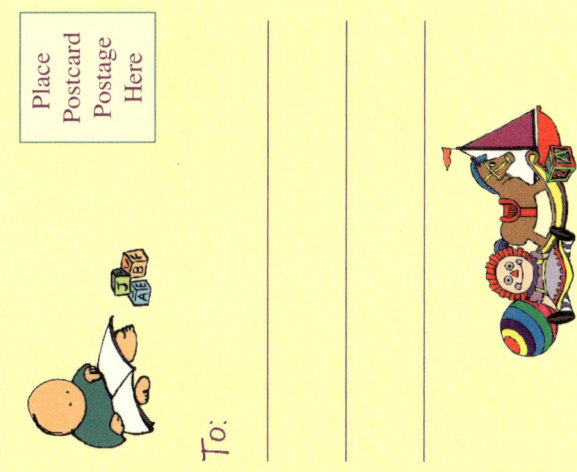

Place Postcard Postage Here

To:

© 1997 Wedding Solutions; San Diego, CA (619) 582-1878

For U.S. Postal Service Use Only

Peel off label, then paste onto the back of your favorite new baby photograph.

Announcing The Arrival Of:

Name:

Date:

Time:

Weight:

Length:

Proud Parents:

"Our New Bundle Of Joy !!"

↓ Peel off label, then paste onto the back of your baby photograph. ↓

Place Postcard Postage Here

↶ Peel off label, then paste onto the back of your favorite new baby photograph. ↷

To:

© 1997 Wedding Solutions; San Diego, CA (619) 582-1878

For U.S. Postal Service Use Only

Announcing The Arrival Of:

Name:

Date:

Time:

Weight:

Length:

Proud Parents:

"Our New Bundle Of Joy!!"

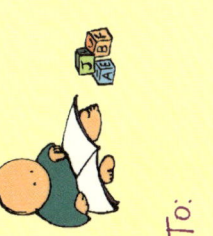

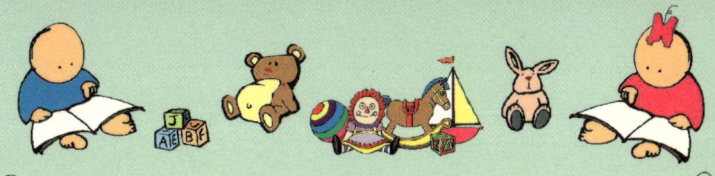

↶ Peel off label, then paste onto the back of your baby photograph. ↷

↶ Peel off label, then paste onto the back of your favorite new baby photograph. ↷

Place Postcard Postage Here

To:

© 1997 Wedding Solutions; San Diego, CA (619) 582-1878

For U.S. Postal Service Use Only

Announcing The Arrival Of:

Name:

Date:

Time:

Weight:

Length:

Proud Parents:

"Our New Bundle Of Joy!!"

↙ Peel off label, then paste onto the back of your baby photograph. ↙

↶ Peel off label, then paste onto the back of your favorite new baby photograph. ↶

Place Postcard Postage Here

To: _____

© 1997 Wedding Solutions; San Diego, CA (619) 582-1878

For U.S. Postal Service Use Only

Announcing The Arrival Of:

Name: _____

Date: _____

Time: _____

Weight: _____

Length: _____

Proud Parents: _____

"Our New Bundle Of Joy !!"

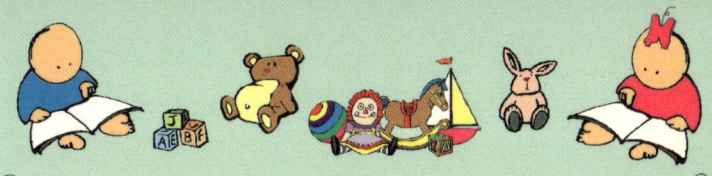

↙ Peel off label, then paste onto the back of your baby photograph. ↙

↶ Peel off label, then paste onto the back of your favorite new baby photograph. ↶

Place Postcard Postage Here

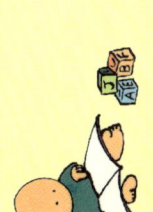

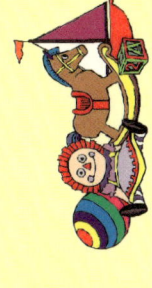

To:

© 1997 Wedding Solutions; San Diego, CA (619) 582-1878

For U.S. Postal Service Use Only

Announcing The Arrival Of:

Name:

Date:

Time:

Weight:

Length:

Proud Parents:

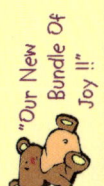

"Our New Bundle Of Joy !!"

↙ Peel off label, then paste onto the back of your baby photograph. ↙

Place Postcard Postage Here

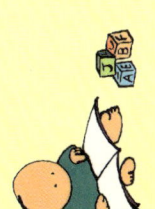

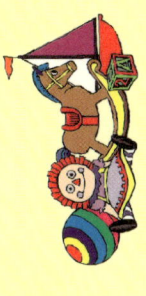

To:

© 1997 Wedding Solutions; San Diego, CA (619) 582-1878

For U.S. Postal Service Use Only

Announcing The Arrival Of:

Name:

Date:

Time:

Weight:

Length:

Proud Parents:

"Our New Bundle Of Joy!!"

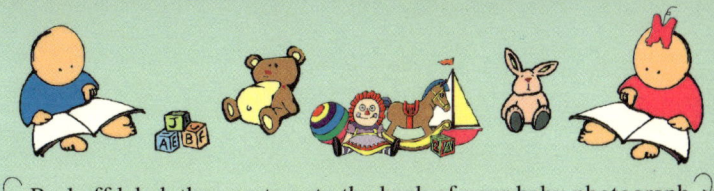

↙ Peel off label, then paste onto the back of your baby photograph. ↙

Place Postcard Postage Here

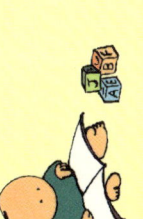

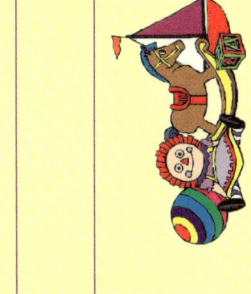

To:

© 1997 Wedding Solutions; San Diego, CA (619) 582-1878

Announcing The Arrival Of:

Name:

Date:

Time:

Weight:

Length:

Proud Parents:

"Our New Bundle Of Joy !!"

For U.S. Postal Service Use Only

↶ Peel off label, then paste onto the back of your favorite new baby photograph. ↷

↶ Peel off label, then paste onto the back of your baby photograph. ↷

Place Postcard Postage Here

To:

© 1997 Wedding Solutions; San Diego, CA (619) 582-1878

For U.S. Postal Service Use Only

↶ Peel off label, then paste onto the back of your favorite new baby photograph. ↷

Announcing The Arrival Of:

Name:

Date:

Time:

Weight:

Length:

Proud Parents:

"Our New Bundle Of Joy !!"

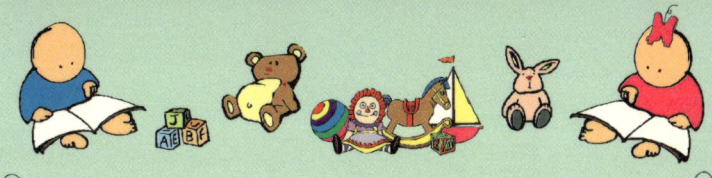

↶ Peel off label, then paste onto the back of your baby photograph. ↷

Place Postcard Postage Here

↷ Peel off label, then paste onto the back of your favorite new baby photograph. ↶

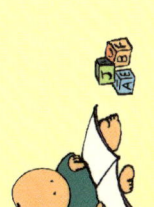

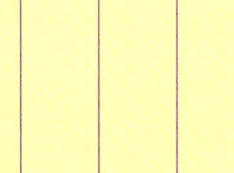

To: _____

© 1997 Wedding Solutions; San Diego, CA (619) 582-1878

For U.S. Postal Service Use Only

Announcing The
Arrival Of:

Name: _____

Date: _____

Time: _____

Weight: _____

Length: _____

Proud Parents: _____

"Our New Bundle Of Joy !!"

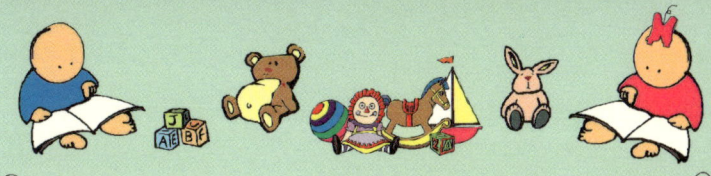

↱ Peel off label, then paste onto the back of your baby photograph. ↰

↱ Peel off label, then paste onto the back of your favorite new baby photograph. ↰

Place Postcard Postage Here

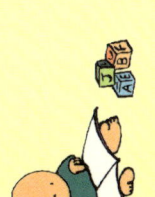

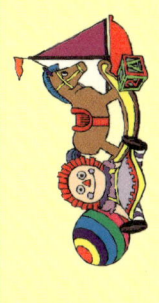

To:

© 1997 Wedding Solutions; San Diego, CA (619) 582-1878

For U.S. Postal Service Use Only

Announcing The Arrival Of:

Name:

Date:

Time:

Weight:

Length:

Proud Parents:

"Our New Bundle Of Joy !!"

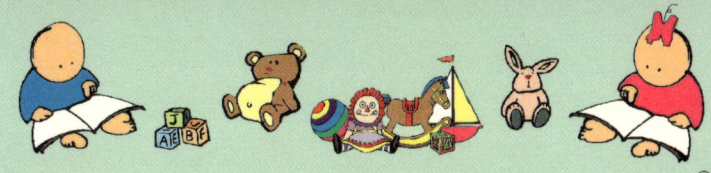

↶ Peel off label, then paste onto the back of your baby photograph. ↷

Place Postcard Postage Here

↶ Peel off label, then paste onto the back of your favorite new baby photograph. ↷

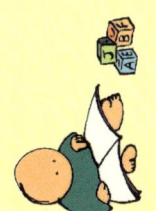

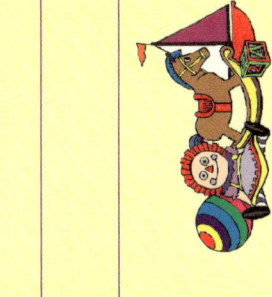

To:

© 1997 Wedding Solutions; San Diego, CA (619) 582-1878

For U.S. Postal Service Use Only

Announcing The Arrival Of:

Name:
Date:
Time:
Weight:
Length:
Proud Parents:

"Our New Bundle Of Joy !!"

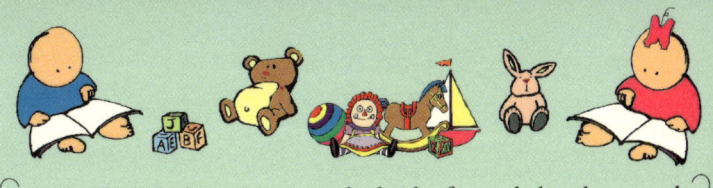

↙ Peel off label, then paste onto the back of your baby photograph. ↙

Place Postcard Postage Here

↶ Peel off label, then paste onto the back of your favorite new baby photograph.

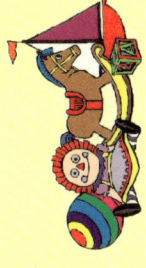

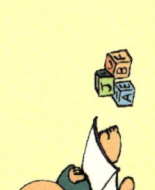

To:

© 1997 Wedding Solutions; San Diego, CA (619) 582-1878

For U.S. Postal Service Use Only

Announcing The Arrival Of:

Name:

Date:

Time:

Weight:

Length:

Proud Parents:

"Our New Bundle Of Joy !!"

↷ Peel off label, then paste onto the back of your baby photograph. ↶

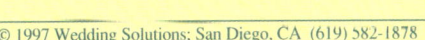
© 1997 Wedding Solutions; San Diego, CA (619) 582-1878

Place Postcard Postage Here

To:

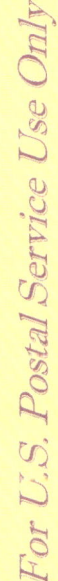
For U.S. Postal Service Use Only

Announcing The Arrival Of:

Name:

Date:

Time:

Weight:

Length:

Proud Parents:

"Our New Bundle Of Joy !!"

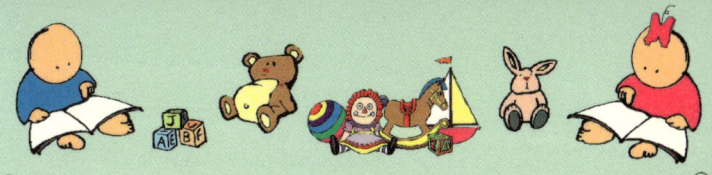

↙ Peel off label, then paste onto the back of your baby photograph. ↙

Place Postcard Postage Here

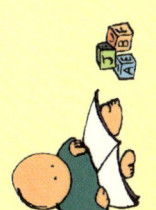

To:

© 1997 Wedding Solutions; San Diego, CA (619) 582-1878

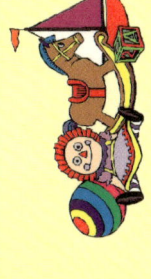

For U.S. Postal Service Use Only

Announcing The
Arrival Of:

Name:

Date:

Time:

Weight:

Length:

Proud Parents:

"Our New Bundle Of Joy !!"

↙ Peel off label, then paste onto the back of your baby photograph. ↘

Place Postcard Postage Here	

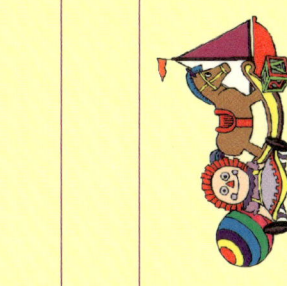

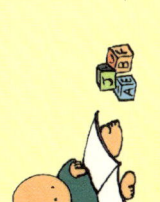

To:

© 1997 Wedding Solutions; San Diego, CA (619) 582-1878

For U.S. Postal Service Use Only

Announcing The Arrival Of:

Name:

Date:

Time:

Weight:

Length:

Proud Parents:

"Our New Bundle Of Joy !!"

↷ Peel off label, then paste onto the back of your baby photograph. ↶

Place Postcard Postage Here

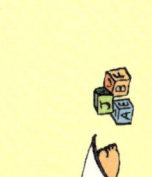

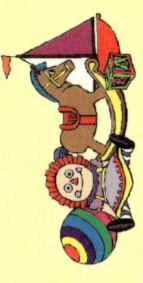

To: _____

© 1997 Wedding Solutions; San Diego, CA (619) 582-1878

For U.S. Postal Service Use Only

Announcing The Arrival Of:

Name: _____
Date: _____
Time: _____
Weight: _____
Length: _____
Proud Parents: _____

"Our New Bundle Of Joy !!"

Peel off label, then paste onto the back of your baby photograph.

Peel off label, then paste onto the back of your favorite new baby photograph.

Place Postcard Postage Here

To:

© 1997 Wedding Solutions; San Diego, CA (619) 582-1878

For U.S. Postal Service Use Only

Announcing The Arrival Of:

Name:

Date:

Time:

Weight:

Length:

Proud Parents:

"Our New Bundle Of Joy !!"

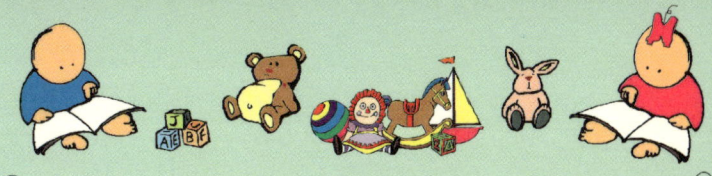

↙ Peel off label, then paste onto the back of your baby photograph. ↙

Place Postcard Postage Here	

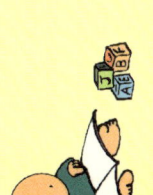
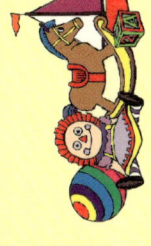

↶ Peel off label, then paste onto the back of your favorite new baby photograph. ↷

To:

© 1997 Wedding Solutions; San Diego, CA (619) 582-1878

For U.S. Postal Service Use Only

Announcing The Arrival Of:

Name:

Date:

Time:

Weight:

Length:

Proud Parents:

"Our New Bundle Of Joy !!"

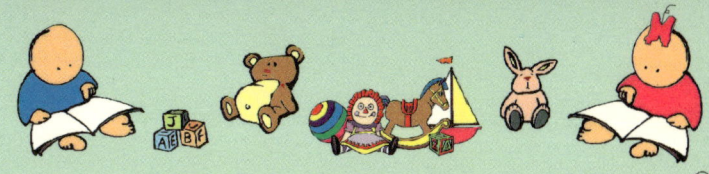

Peel off label, then paste onto the back of your baby photograph.

Place Postcard Postage Here

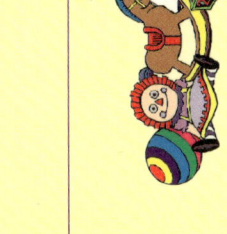

To:

© 1997 Wedding Solutions; San Diego, CA (619) 582-1878

Peel off label, then paste onto the back of your favorite new baby photograph.

Announcing The Arrival Of:

Name:
Date:
Time:
Weight:
Length:
Proud Parents:

For U.S. Postal Service Use Only

"Our New Bundle Of Joy!!"

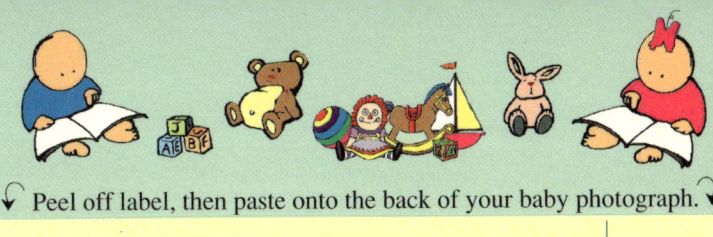

↓ Peel off label, then paste onto the back of your baby photograph. ↓

↰ Peel off label, then paste onto the back of your favorite new baby photograph. ↰

Place Postcard Postage Here

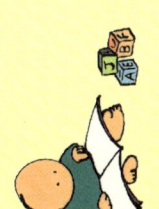

To:

© 1997 Wedding Solutions; San Diego, CA (619) 582-1878

For U.S. Postal Service Use Only

Announcing The Arrival Of:

Name:

Date:

Time:

Weight:

Length:

Proud Parents:

"Our New Bundle Of Joy !!"